STREP THROAT

SIMPLE MEANS OF TREATING STREP THROAT

DR. J. WALLER

Contents

Introduction

The tonsils and throat are the main areas affected by strep throat, which is a bacterial illness. Streptococcus pyogenes, a member of the group A Streptococcus bacteria, is the source of this prevalent infection. Although it can affect anyone at any age, strep throat is particularly contagious and is most commonly found in children and adolescents.

Crucial details regarding strep throat consist of:

Reasons:

Streptococcus pyogenes is the organism that causes strep throat. When an infected individual coughs or sneezes, respiratory droplets are released into the air, and surfaces contaminated with the bacterium can also become contaminated.

Signs:

A sore throat, trouble swallowing, fever, headache, and red or white patches on the tonsils are typical signs of strep throat. Coughing or runny nose may not accompany strep throat, in contrast to viral sore throats.

Contagious Characteristics:

People who have strep throat are highly contagious and can infect others through close contact. Practicing good hygiene, such as cleaning your hands after handling a sneeze or cough, can help stop the spread of the illness.

A quick strep test or throat swab can be used by a medical expert to diagnose strep throat. Since antibiotics work well to treat strep throat but not viral infections, this is crucial in differentiating it from other causes of sore throat.

Therapy:

Doctors administer antibiotics, most often amoxicillin or penicillin, to treat strep throat. Even if symptoms get better, it's still important to finish the entire course of antibiotics to avoid problems and lower the chance of recurrence.

Problems:

Complications from strep throat may include rheumatic fever, post-streptococcal glomerulonephritis, or infection spreading to other areas of the body if treatment is not received.

Avoidance:

The spread of the virus can be stopped by maintaining proper cleanliness, avoiding close contact with sick people, and getting medical care as soon as strep throat symptoms appear.

Separation:

When someone is diagnosed with strep throat, they are frequently told not to go to work or school until they have been taking antibiotics for at least 24 hours in order to minimize the chance of infection spread.

In most cases, strep throat is curable and controllable with the right medical care. Getting medical help as soon as possible, finishing the recommended course of antibiotics, and adopting preventive measures can all help patients heal more quickly and experience fewer difficulties.

CHAPTER ONE

Recognizing Symptoms

For an early diagnosis and course of treatment, it is imperative to recognize the symptoms of strep throat. Certain symptoms are particularly specific to strep throat, even if others may also be present in other respiratory illnesses. Typical signs and symptoms include of:

Throat Pain:

A sharp, acute sore throat is the typical first symptom of strep throat. When swallowing, the pain could be very noticeable.

White Patches on Red Tonsils:

The tonsils may have streaks or areas of white or yellowish color on their surface, and they may appear red and swollen.

Temperature spike:

One common sign of strep throat is fever. The body can heat up to more than 38.3 degrees Celsius, or 101 degrees Fahrenheit.

Headache:

Headaches: People who have strep throat frequently get mild to moderate headaches.

Enlarged lymph nodes

The infection may cause the neck's lymph nodes, or glands, to swell and become tender.

Having Trouble Swallowing:

People who have strep throat may feel pain and have trouble swallowing due to the inflammation in their throat.

Rash

A delicate red rash called "scarlet fever" may appear in certain people. Usually beginning on the chest and belly, this rash can extend to other parts of the body.

Vomiting and nauseous:

Certain people with strep throat, particularly children, may feel queasy or throw up.

It's crucial to remember that compared to viral respiratory illnesses like the flu or the common cold, strep throat symptoms like congestion, coughing, and runny nose are less frequent. If these signs and symptoms are present, a viral rather than bacterial etiology may be suspected.

Seeking medical assistance is advised if someone exhibits the symptoms of strep throat, particularly if they are severe or persistent. To confirm the diagnosis, a medical expert may do a quick strep test or a throat swab. Antibiotic treatment must begin as soon as possible in order to relieve symptoms, avoid complications, and lower the chance of infection transmission.

Reasons and Mode of Transmission

The bacteria Streptococcus pyogenes, sometimes referred to as group A Streptococcus, is the cause of strep throat. The virus is extremely contagious and can spread in a number of ways, including:

Direct Communication:

The most common way for strep throat to spread is through direct touch between people. This can happen when someone who is infected coughs or sneezes, sending respiratory droplets that are contaminated with germs into the surrounding air.

Airborne Transmission:

In close proximity to an infected person, respiratory droplets containing the Streptococcus pyogenes bacteria can be inhaled. This is particularly typical in cramped or congested areas.

Contacting Polluted Surfaces:

The spread of strep throat can occur when an infected surface or object comes into contact with the mouth, nose, or eyes after being touched.

Exchanging Individual Goods:

The germs can spread by sharing personal objects with an infected person, such as cups, towels, or cutlery.

Not Enough Hand Sanitization

The spread of strep throat can be aided by poor hand hygiene, such as not washing hands frequently with soap and water.

Intimate Contact:

The risk of transmission is increased by close contact with an infected person, particularly in homes, schools, or workplaces.

State of Carrier:

Some people might not exhibit any signs of strep throat, but they could nonetheless be carriers of Streptococcus pyogenes. The germs can still spread to other people through carriers.

Though it can afflict people of any age, it's crucial to remember that strep throat is more common in children and teens. Because the strep throat germs may live on surfaces for a short time, strep throat is highly contagious.

It is important to maintain proper hygiene and take preventative measures to stop the spread of strep throat. These precautions include:

Regular Handwashing: Always wash your hands well with soap and water, especially after using the restroom, sneezing, coughing, or coming into contact with potentially contaminated surfaces.

Minimize Close Contact: Especially during the contagious period, avoid close contact with people who are known to have strep throat.

Respiratory Hygiene: To stop the release of respiratory droplets when coughing or sneezing, cover your mouth and nose with a tissue or your elbow.

Not Sharing Personal Items: Avoid sharing cups, cutlery, or towels with anyone who might be contaminated.

Fast Medical Attention: If you start experiencing strep throat symptoms, get help right away. Antibiotic therapy administered promptly can shorten the duration of symptoms and stop the illness from spreading.

By following these preventive steps, communities and households can reduce their risk of contracting or spreading strep throat.

Identification

The diagnosis of strep throat is usually made using a combination of laboratory testing and clinical assessment. Medical practitioners employ many techniques to ascertain if the infection is being caused by Streptococcus pyogenes bacterium. Typical diagnostic techniques consist of:

Throat Culture:

Gathering a swab sample from the tonsils and back of the throat is necessary for a throat culture. After the sample is taken, it is grown in a lab to determine whether Streptococcus pyogenes bacteria are present. Although this procedure yields accurate answers, the final decision may take one to two days.

Quick Strep Test:

A faster diagnostic technique with minutes-long results is the rapid strep test. A sample is taken using a throat swab, and Streptococcus pyogenes antigens are found in the sample. Compared to a throat culture, this test can have a little greater false-negative rate despite being quicker.

Clinical Assessment:

To arrive at a preliminary diagnosis, medical practitioners evaluate the patient's physical examination results, medical history, and symptoms. Frequent symptoms of strep throat include fever, swollen tonsils, white or yellowish patches on the tonsils, and an abrupt, intense sore throat.

Elimination of viral origins:

It's critical to differentiate strep throat from viral sore throat reasons, such as the flu or the common cold, because the former is a bacterial infection. If there are no usual viral symptoms, including coughing and runny nose, then a bacterial source could be the reason.

Evaluation of Symptoms:

Based on particular symptoms, the probability of having strep throat can occasionally be determined using the Centor criteria, a set of clinical recommendations. Fever, tonsillar exudates (pus on the tonsils), painful and swollen anterior cervical lymph nodes, and a cough are among the requirements.

It's critical that people with symptoms that could indicate strep throat get medical assistance in order to receive an accurate diagnosis and appropriate treatment. Antibiotic treatment must begin as soon as possible in order to relieve symptoms, avoid complications, and lower the chance of infection transmission.

It is not advisable to self-diagnose based only on symptoms because similar symptoms can be present in other illnesses. If strep throat is the cause of the symptoms, a medical practitioner will accurately establish it by a mix of clinical judgment and diagnostic procedures.

Strategies for Treatment

Antibiotics are the mainstay of treatment for strep throat since they eradicate the Streptococcus pyogenes bacterial infection. Furthermore, supportive actions can aid in symptom relief and rehabilitation. The following are the main strep throat treatment methods:

Antibiotics:

For treating strep throat, antibiotics like amoxicillin and penicillin are the mainstay. These drugs reduce the length of the sickness and efficiently eradicate the Streptococcus pyogenes germs. Even if symptoms subside before taking the last pill, it's imperative to finish the entire course of antibiotics as directed by the doctor.

CHAPTER TWO

Pain Management:

Acetaminophen (Tylenol) and ibuprofen (Advil, Motrin) are two over-the-counter pain medications that can help lessen strep throat-related pain, fever, and inflammation. Observe the suggested dose guidelines.

Throat sprays or lozenges:

Throat sprays or lozenges with numbing ingredients can offer momentary respite from the sensations of a sore throat. These, however, are only palliative measures; the underlying infection is not treated by them.

Drinking plenty of water

It's critical to maintain adequate hydration when suffering from strep throat. Staying hydrated and relieving sore throats can be achieved by consuming lots of water, herbal teas, and clear broths.

Relax:

Resting enough is necessary for the body to heal from the infection. Rest well and steer clear of physically demanding activities that could impair your immune system's capacity to combat microorganisms.

Using a Humidifier:

By adding moisture to the air in the bedroom, a humidifier helps ease breathing difficulties and soothe throat irritation.

Separation and Proactive Steps:

When coughing or sneezing, people with strep throat should cover their mouth and nose as part of basic respiratory hygiene. To stop the infection from spreading, they should also keep their distance from other people for at least 24 hours after beginning antibiotic treatment.

Observation

Keep any follow-up appointments that the doctor recommends in order to make sure the infection has been successfully treated. If antibiotic treatment doesn't alleviate the symptoms, more testing might be required.

For an accurate diagnosis and course of treatment, it's critical that those who feel they may have strep throat seek medical help as soon as possible. Antibiotics should be started as soon as possible to assist shorten the duration of symptoms, avoid complications, and lower the chance of infection transmission. Adhering to supportive measures can also improve comfort and speed up the healing process.

Natural Treatments and Symptom Control

Although the main course of therapy for strep throat is antibiotics, there are a number of do-at-home cures and symptom management techniques that can ease discomfort and aid in the healing process. The following are some natural cures for strep throat:

Drinking plenty of water

Make sure you stay hydrated by consuming lots of water, herbal teas, and clear broths. Staying hydrated helps avoid dehydration and ease sore throats.

Warm Salt Rinse:

Gargling with warm seawater might help lessen inflammation and ease sore throats. Gargle with a solution made from one teaspoon salt and warm water many times a day.

Hard candies or throat lozenges:

Symptoms of sore throat might be momentarily relieved by sucking on hard candy or throat lozenges. Select products that have calming components such as honey or menthol.

Using a Humidifier:

By adding moisture to the air in the bedroom, a humidifier can help reduce throat discomfort and improve breathing comfort.

Relax:

Give your body enough time to relax and heal. Steer clear of demanding tasks and get enough sleep.

Nonprescription Painkillers:

Pain, fever, and inflammation can all be decreased with over-the-counter pain medicines such ibuprofen (Advil, Motrin) or acetaminophen (Tylenol). Observe the suggested dose guidelines.

Remain Warm:

Stay warm, particularly if you're feeling chilly. If you want to keep your body temperature comfortable, use blankets and layers of clothing.

Herbal Teas:

Herbal teas with chamomile, honey, and ginger can be calming and help ease sore throats.

Soft Meals:

Choose for foods that are soft and simple to swallow, including mashed potatoes, soups, and broths. Steer clear of acidic or spicy foods that can irritate the throat.

Steer clear of irritants:

Avoid smoke and other allergens that might exacerbate sore throats. If you smoke, think about cutting back on your tobacco use.

It's crucial to remember that although these natural treatments can lessen discomfort and help control symptoms, they cannot take the place of medical professionals' prescription antibiotics. To eradicate the bacterial infection causing strep throat, antibiotics are necessary.

Seeking medical assistance is advised for additional evaluation and appropriate management if symptoms do not improve with home remedies, or if the severity of the infection is a concern.

Although strep throat is usually curable, complications or untreated cases may result in more significant health problems. It's critical to be aware of potential side effects and to get help if you have any particular indications or symptoms. Among the potential strep throat complications are:

Fever with Rheumatism:

A rare but dangerous side effect of not getting enough treatment for strep throat is rheumatic fever. The nervous system, skin, joints, and heart could all be impacted. Rheumatoid arthritis fever can be avoided with prompt antibiotic treatment.

Glomerulonephritis caused by streptococci:

This illness, which can follow a strep throat infection, is characterized by inflammation of the kidneys. It could cause symptoms like edema, elevated blood pressure, and adjustments to urine production.

Abscess peritonsillar:

A pus-filled mass that develops close to the tonsils is called a peritonsillar abscess. It may result in a muffled voice, excruciating throat pain, and trouble swallowing. Antibiotic therapy and drainage are frequently necessary.

Red Fever:

A bacterial infection known as scarlet fever can strike people who have strep throat. It requires antibiotics for therapy and is characterized by a red rash, fever, and a "strawberry tongue."

Infections of the ears:

Ear infections can occasionally result from strep throat, especially in young children. An ear infection may be indicated by ear pain, fluid discharge, and hearing loss.

Sinus inflammation:

If strep throat is left untreated, a consequence that might arise is sinusitis, or inflammation of the sinuses. Sinus pressure, nasal congestion, and facial pain are among the symptoms.

Abscesses:

Abscesses may develop in the throat or its surrounding tissues as a result of the illness. Antibiotic therapy and drainage may be necessary for abscesses.

It is imperative that you get medical help if you encounter any of the following:

- Severe or chronic throat pain
- Breathing or swallowing difficulties
- Elevated fever that does not go down with therapy
- Persistent symptoms that don't get better upon taking antibiotics
- emergence of fresh signs or issues

Even if symptoms get better before taking the last dose of antibiotics, it's imperative to continue the entire course of treatment if strep throat is identified. This lowers the chance of problems and recurrence.

Contact a healthcare provider right away for additional assessment and suitable management if there are worries about the infection's course or the emergence of consequences. Preventing and managing potential problems linked to strep throat necessitates early management.

Preventive Actions

Taking preventive action can lessen the chance of contracting and transmitting strep throat. The following are a few methods to reduce the chance of getting strep throat:

CHAPTER THREE

Proper Handling Techniques:

Hands should be periodically cleaned with soap and water, particularly after sneezing, coughing, or coming into close contact with sick people. Keeping hands clean aids in halting the spread of bacteria.

Breathing Hygiene:

When sneezing or coughing, cover your mouth and nose with your elbow or a tissue to stop the spread of bacteria-laden respiratory droplets.

Steer clear of close contact:

Reduce your close contact with those who have been diagnosed or suspected of having strep throat. This is especially crucial during the infectious window, which lasts for at least 24 hours following the initiation of antibiotic therapy.

Not Exchanging Private Objects:

Avoid sharing glasses, cutlery, water bottles, and other personal objects with people who might be contaminated.

Sustain a Healthy Way of Life:

A balanced diet, frequent exercise, and enough sleep are all components of a healthy lifestyle that enhance immune system performance.

Encourage proper oral hygiene:

To lower the danger of bacterial growth in the mouth, practice good oral hygiene by brushing and flossing your teeth on a regular basis.

Instruct and Promote Good Hygiene in Children:

Teach kids the value of cleaning their hands, covering their mouths and noses when they cough or sneeze, and refraining from sharing personal objects.

Quick Medical Attention:

When someone experiences sore throat symptoms, they should get medical help right once to ensure a correct diagnosis and course of therapy. Antibiotics taken at an early stage can shorten the duration of symptoms and stop the infection from spreading.

Remain Up to Date:

Learn about the signs and treatments of strep throat. People who are aware of the illness are better able to take the necessary safety measures and, when necessary, seek prompt medical assistance.

Ensure that the Environment Is Clean:

To lower the chance of bacterial transmission, regularly clean and disinfect frequently touched areas including light switches, doorknobs, and shared electronics.

It's crucial to remember that while taking these precautions can help lower the chance of developing strep throat, total prevention may not always be achievable. People who experience recurring or ongoing symptoms, or who are in close proximity to someone who has been verified to have the illness, ought to consult a physician for assessment and proper treatment.

CONCLUSION

In conclusion, Streptococcus pyogenes, also referred to as group A Streptococcus, is the bacterial infection that causes strep throat. The tonsils and throat are the main areas affected, resulting in symptoms like fever, painful throat, and difficulty swallowing. Highly contagious, strep throat can spread by contact with contaminated surfaces or by respiratory droplets.

Rapid strep tests and throat cultures are two examples of the laboratory tests used in conjunction with clinical evaluation to make the diagnosis. Antibiotics must be used promptly and appropriately to treat the infection in order to lessen symptoms, avoid complications, and lower the chance of spreading to other people.

Using throat lozenges, staying hydrated, and getting enough sleep are examples of home remedies and supportive measures that can help control symptoms and improve comfort while recovering. These actions, however, need to support doctor-prescribed antibiotic therapy rather than take its place.

Although they are uncommon, rheumatic fever, post-streptococcal glomerulonephritis, and abscess formation are possible complications of strep throat. It is imperative to seek medical assistance for symptoms that are severe or persistent in order to prevent and manage any problems.

Good hygiene habits, respiratory hygiene, and avoiding close contact with sick people are examples of preventive actions that can help lower the chance of contracting and spreading strep throat.

To summarize, prompt diagnosis, suitable antibiotic therapy, and supportive care can expedite the healing process and reduce the likelihood of complications associated with strep throat. People who exhibit symptoms that could indicate they have strep throat should consult a doctor for a full assessment and customized treatment.

THE END